100% NATURAL REMEDY 4 FEMALE Reproductive System Disorders

Simplified Guide On How To Treat & Prevent Female Reproductive System Disorders Like; Infertility, PCOS, POI, Vaginitis, Fibroids, Abnormal Uterine Bleeding, Endometriosis, Cervical Cancer, Interstitial Cystitis (IC), Etc.

MRS. VERA JACOB

Copyright Notice.

Contents

INTRODUCTION

Welcome to a journey of fertility, fruitfulness, and a happy marriage life packed with the secrets of becoming a gracious mother, enjoying the joy of motherhood, and an empowerment program to take full charge of your reproductive system's health.

In this book titled, "100% NATURAL REMEDY 4 FEMALE Reproductive System Disorders." The author will walk you through the wisdom of nature and the latest insights in holistic health to navigate the realms of botanical remedies, nutritional harmony, and empowering practices to nurture your reproductive system back to its natural state of balance, prevent, manage, and treat any form or types of female reproductive system disorder, such as; Infertility, PCOS, POI, Vaginitis, Fibroids, Abnormal Uterine Bleeding, Endometriosis, Cervical Cancer, Interstitial

Cystitis (IC), Etc.

This book won't only help you to be a mother and live a healthy life but can help you to prevent, manage and treat any form or type of female reproductive system disorder, give you access to a transformative power of nature's remedies to reclaim vitality, restore harmony, and bloom with radiant health.

You want to keep reading and be completely free from any form of female reproductive system disorder, HIT THE BUY BUTTON NOW!

CHAPTER ONE
What are Female Reproductive System Disorders?

The female reproductive system is susceptible to various disorders that can negatively affect the reproductive organs and hormonal balance in women. These conditions can range from mild to severe and may affect fertility, menstrual cycles, hormonal balance, and overall reproductive health. Some of the common female reproductive system disorders are:

1. **Polycystic Ovary Syndrome (PCOS):** A hormonal disorder causing enlarged ovaries with small cysts on the outer edges. It can lead to irregular periods, infertility, and hormonal imbalances.

2. **Primary Ovarian Insufficiency (POI):** Formerly known as premature ovarian failure, POI involves the

loss of normal ovarian function before the age of 40, leading to irregular periods, infertility, and hormonal disruptions.

3. **Infertility:** Inability to conceive after a year of regular, unprotected intercourse. This can be due to various factors, including hormonal imbalances, ovulation issues, anatomical problems, or underlying medical conditions.

4. **Vaginitis:** Inflammation of the vagina often caused by infections, changes in vaginal pH, or reactions to irritants. It leads to discomfort, itching, discharge, and sometimes pain during intercourse.

5. **Fibroids**: Noncancerous growths in the uterus that can cause pain, heavy menstrual bleeding, pelvic pressure, and sometimes fertility issues.

6. **Abnormal Uterine Bleeding:** Irregular, heavy, or prolonged bleeding outside the normal menstrual cycle, often caused by hormonal imbalances, uterine fibroids, or structural issues.

7. **Endometriosis:** A condition where tissue similar to the lining of the uterus grows outside the uterus, causing pain, heavy periods, and infertility.

8. **Cervical Cancer:** Cancer that develops in the cervix, often linked to the human papillomavirus (HPV) infection.

9. **Interstitial Cystitis:** Also known as painful bladder syndrome, it's a chronic condition causing bladder pain and pressure, frequent urination, and pelvic discomfort.

These disorders can significantly impact a woman's quality

of life, reproductive health, and emotional well-being. Treatment approaches often include a combination of medication, lifestyle changes, surgical interventions, and in many cases, natural remedies aimed at managing symptoms and promoting overall health.

Understanding PCOS

Polycystic Ovary Syndrome (PCOS) presents a labyrinth of complexities, affecting millions of individuals worldwide, particularly those assigned female at birth. This multifaceted endocrine disorder involves hormonal imbalances, metabolic irregularities, and reproductive challenges, forming a complex web of symptoms and implications that extend far beyond the physical realm.

At its core, PCOS involves an interplay of hormones, primarily androgens like testosterone, and the disruption of insulin production or utilization, leading to irregular menstrual cycles, ovarian cysts, weight fluctuations, and difficulties with fertility. However, its impact isn't limited to these manifestations alone; it often intertwines with emotional, psychological, and societal aspects, posing significant challenges for those affected.

One of the perplexing aspects of PCOS is its heterogeneity. No two individuals experience the exact same array of symptoms or severity. This diversity makes diagnosis and treatment a convoluted journey. Some may battle weight gain and insulin resistance, while others grapple with severe acne, hair loss, or emotional distress. This variability underscores the importance of personalized care and treatment plans tailored to the specific needs of each individual.

The emotional toll of PCOS cannot be overstated. The

physical manifestations often intersect with body image issues, depression, anxiety, and a sense of frustration stemming from the lack of control over one's body. Societal pressures and misconceptions further compound these emotional struggles, fostering feelings of isolation and inadequacy.

Navigating PCOS requires a multidisciplinary approach. Medical professionals, including endocrinologists, gynecologists, nutritionists, and mental health specialists, play pivotal roles in managing the syndrome. Lifestyle modifications, such as dietary changes, exercise, and stress management, often form the cornerstone of treatment. Medications targeting specific symptoms or hormone regulation might be prescribed, along with fertility treatments for those aiming to conceive.

Education and advocacy are crucial in addressing the

complexities of PCOS. Raising awareness about the syndrome, debunking myths, and fostering a supportive community can empower individuals affected by PCOS to seek proper care, find solidarity, and advocate for their needs within healthcare systems.

Furthermore, research into PCOS remains essential for better understanding its underlying mechanisms and developing more effective treatments. Advancements in scientific understanding and medical technologies offer hope for improved management and possibly even prevention in the future.

Ultimately, navigating the intricacies of PCOS demands patience, resilience, and a holistic approach. It's about acknowledging the multifaceted nature of the syndrome, embracing individual journeys, and fostering a supportive environment that empowers those affected to manage their symptoms and lead fulfilling lives despite its complexities.

Symptoms and Diagnostic Approaches

Polycystic Ovary Syndrome (PCOS) is a complex hormonal disorder that can manifest in various ways, and its diagnosis relies on a combination of symptoms, physical examinations, and medical tests.

Symptoms:

1. **Irregular Periods:** Often one of the initial signs, characterized by infrequent, irregular, or prolonged menstrual cycles.

2. **Excess Androgens:** High levels of male hormones (androgens) can lead to symptoms like acne, excessive facial or body hair (hirsutism), and male-pattern baldness.

3. **Ovarian Cysts:** While not always present, the condition is named for the appearance of small, fluid-filled sacs on the ovaries.

4. **Metabolic Issues:** Insulin resistance, which may result in weight gain, difficulty losing weight, and increased risk of type 2 diabetes.

5. **Fertility Problems:** PCOS is a leading cause of infertility due to irregular ovulation or failure to ovulate regularly.

Diagnostic Approaches:

1. **Medical History and Physical Examination:** A doctor will review symptoms, and menstrual history, and perform a physical examination to check for signs of excess hair growth, acne, and weight issues.

2. **Blood Tests:** Hormone level assessment, particularly androgens (testosterone), estrogen, LH (luteinizing hormone), FSH (follicle-stimulating hormone), and insulin levels.

3. **Pelvic Exam and Ultrasound:** An ultrasound is conducted to examine the ovaries for the presence of cysts or enlarged ovaries.

4. **Exclusion of other conditions:** Other conditions with similar symptoms, like thyroid disorders or adrenal gland problems, may be ruled out.

Diagnostic Criteria:

The Rotterdam criteria, often used for diagnosis, require the presence of at least two out of three criteria:

i. Irregular periods or lack of ovulation.

ii. Clinical or biochemical signs of high androgens (like excess hair growth or elevated testosterone).

iii. Polycystic ovaries visible on ultrasound.

Challenges in Diagnosis:

Diagnosing PCOS can be challenging due to its varied presentation and the overlap of symptoms with other conditions. Additionally, not all individuals with PCOS will have ovarian cysts, and some may have cysts without exhibiting the typical symptoms.

Early diagnosis and proper management are crucial in PCOS to prevent long-term complications, such as infertility, metabolic syndrome, and cardiovascular disease.

A multidisciplinary approach involving gynecologists, endocrinologists, dieticians, and mental health professionals is often necessary to provide comprehensive care tailored to individual needs.

Natural Remedies for Managing PCOS

Natural remedies and lifestyle changes can complement traditional treatments in managing Polycystic Ovary Syndrome (PCOS). While they might not cure PCOS, they can help alleviate symptoms and improve overall well-being. Here are some strategies:

Diet Modifications:

1. **Balanced Diet:** Focus on whole foods, fruits, vegetables, lean proteins, and complex carbohydrates to manage insulin levels.

2. **Low Glycemic Index (GI) Foods:** Choose foods that don't cause rapid spikes in blood sugar levels, like whole grains, legumes, and non-starchy vegetables.

3. **Limit Sugar and Processed Foods:** Minimize intake of sugary snacks, processed foods, and sweetened beverages.

4. **Healthy Fats:** Incorporate sources of healthy fats like avocados, nuts, seeds, and fatty fish, which can help regulate hormone production.

Regular Exercise:

1. **Aerobic Exercise:** Regular aerobic activity helps improve insulin sensitivity and manage weight, reducing the impact of PCOS symptoms.

2. **Strength Training:** Building muscle can also aid in managing insulin resistance.

Stress Management:

1. **Mindfulness and Relaxation Techniques:** Practices like yoga, meditation, deep breathing exercises, or mindfulness can help reduce stress, which can exacerbate PCOS symptoms.

2. **Adequate Sleep:** Aim for consistent, restorative sleep to regulate hormonal balance.

Herbal Supplements:

1. **Cinnamon:** May help improve insulin sensitivity and regulate menstrual cycles.

2. **Inositol:** Some studies suggest inositol supplements can aid in improving insulin sensitivity and ovarian function.

3. **Spearmint Tea:** It may help reduce excess hair growth (hirsutism) by lowering androgen levels.

Weight Management:

1. **Healthy Weight:** Maintaining a healthy weight can significantly improve symptoms of PCOS, particularly insulin resistance.

2. **Avoid Crash Diets:** Rapid weight loss methods can negatively impact hormone levels; focus on sustainable, gradual changes.

Regular Monitoring and Support:

1. **Track Symptoms:** Keep a journal to monitor how diet, exercise, and stress management impact symptoms.

2. **Support Groups:** Joining support groups or seeking guidance from healthcare professionals experienced in managing PCOS can provide valuable insights and support.

Caution and Consultation:

While these natural remedies can be beneficial, it's essential to consult healthcare professionals before starting any new regimen, especially if you're considering supplements or major dietary changes. PCOS varies widely among individuals, so personalized advice is crucial.

Integrating these natural remedies into a comprehensive treatment plan, including medical interventions, when necessary, can enhance the management of PCOS and improve overall quality of life.

CHAPTER TWO
Understanding and Decoding POI (Primary Ovarian Insufficiency)

Primary Ovarian Insufficiency (POI), also known as premature ovarian failure or early menopause, is a condition where the ovaries stop functioning normally before the age of 40 (forty). This leads to a decrease in estrogen levels and can result in menstrual irregularities, infertility, and various hormonal imbalances.

Causes of POI:

1. **Genetic Factors:** Some cases of POI have a genetic component, while others may occur sporadically.

2. **Autoimmune Disorders:** When the body's immune system mistakenly attacks the ovaries, it can lead to their dysfunction.

3. **Chromosomal Abnormalities:** Certain genetic conditions, such as Turner syndrome, can be associated with POI.

4. **Chemotherapy or Radiation Therapy:** Cancer treatments can damage the ovaries, leading to premature failure.

5. **Environmental Factors:** Exposure to toxins or environmental factors might contribute to early ovarian failure.

Symptoms and Diagnosis

Symptoms:

1. **Irregular or Absent Periods:** This is a primary sign, where menstruation becomes irregular or stops completely.

2. **Hot Flashes:** Similar to menopausal symptoms, women with POI may experience hot flashes and night sweats.

3. **Vaginal Dryness:** Decreased estrogen levels can lead to vaginal dryness, impacting sexual health.

4. **Difficulty Conceiving:** Infertility or difficulty conceiving due to a lack of ovulation can be a significant symptom.

Diagnosis:

1. **Blood Tests:** Hormone tests measuring levels of estrogen, FSH (follicle-stimulating hormone), LH (luteinizing hormone), and AMH (anti-Müllerian hormone) can indicate ovarian function.

2. **Pelvic Exam and Ultrasound:** An examination may be performed to check for physical signs of ovarian abnormalities.

3. **Genetic Testing:** In some cases, genetic testing might be recommended, especially if there's a suspected genetic cause.

Management and Treatment:

1. **Hormone Replacement Therapy (HRT):** Estrogen and sometimes progesterone replacement can help manage symptoms and prevent complications like osteoporosis.

2. **Fertility Treatments:** In some cases, assisted reproductive techniques such as in vitro fertilization (IVF) may be considered if fertility is desired.

3. **Emotional Support and Counseling:** Coping with the emotional impact of POI, such as fertility

concerns and hormonal changes, often requires support and counseling.

Challenges and Considerations:

- **Fertility Concerns:** POI can affect fertility, so women diagnosed with POI often face emotional challenges related to family planning.

- **Long-term Health Risks:** Estrogen deficiency can increase the risk of osteoporosis and heart disease, among other health concerns.

- **Psychological Impact:** Dealing with the diagnosis and its impact on fertility can lead to emotional distress, requiring support and counseling.

Managing POI involves a multidisciplinary approach, including gynecologists, endocrinologists, and mental health professionals. While it presents challenges, understanding and early intervention can help mitigate symptoms and improve the overall quality of life for individuals affected by POI.

Natural Approaches for Coping with POI

Coping with Primary Ovarian Insufficiency (POI) can be challenging, but integrating natural approaches alongside medical treatments can help manage symptoms and improve overall well-being. Below are some natural strategies that you can consider:

Diet and Nutrition:

1. **Calcium and Vitamin D:** Incorporate foods rich in calcium (such as dairy, leafy greens, and fortified foods) and vitamin D (like fatty fish, egg yolks, and sunlight exposure) to support bone health.

2. **Phytoestrogens:** Foods like soy products, flaxseeds, and legumes contain phytoestrogens, which may mildly mimic estrogen effects and alleviate some symptoms.

Stress Management:

1. **Mindfulness and Relaxation Techniques:** Practices like yoga, meditation, or deep breathing exercises can help reduce stress and improve overall well-being.

2. **Support Groups or Counseling:** Joining support groups or seeking counseling can provide emotional support and coping strategies.

Regular Exercise:

1. **Weight-Bearing Exercises:** Engage in weight-bearing exercises (such as walking, dancing, or

weightlifting) to support bone health and improve overall fitness.

2. **Yoga or Tai Chi:** These activities can promote relaxation, flexibility, and stress reduction.

Herbal Supplements and Alternative Therapies:

1. **Black Cohosh:** Some women find relief from symptoms like hot flashes with black cohosh supplements, although results vary.

2. **Acupuncture:** This traditional Chinese therapy might help manage symptoms like hot flashes and mood swings in some individuals.

Lifestyle Modifications:

1. **Adequate Sleep:** Prioritize good sleep hygiene to support overall health and hormone regulation.

2. **Avoiding Toxins:** Minimize exposure to environmental toxins and chemicals that may disrupt hormone balance.

Regular Monitoring and Self-Care:

1. **Track Symptoms:** Keeping a symptom diary can help identify patterns and triggers, allowing better management.

2. **Self-Care Practices:** Engage in activities that promote relaxation and self-care, such as reading, hobbies, or spending time outdoors.

POI can impact various aspects of life, including fertility and emotional well-being. Integrating these natural approaches into a comprehensive care plan, alongside medical treatments and support, can enhance the management of POI and improve quality of life.

CHAPTER THREE
Fertility Challenges: Infertility and Solutions

Infertility can be emotionally distressing and complex, affecting individuals and couples trying to conceive. Various factors contribute to fertility challenges:

1. **Ovulatory Issues:** Conditions like PCOS or POI can affect ovulation, leading to irregular or absent menstrual cycles.

2. **Male Factor Infertility:** Problems with sperm quality, quantity, or delivery can hinder conception.

3. **Tubal Issues:** Blockages or damage to the fallopian tubes can impede the egg's journey to the uterus.

4. **Uterine or Structural Issues:** Abnormalities in the uterus or cervix might impact fertility.

5. **Age-related Factors:** Fertility declines with age, particularly for women, due to decreased egg quantity and quality.

Solutions and Approaches:

1. **Medical Intervention:**

- **Fertility Treatments:** Assisted reproductive technologies like in vitro fertilization (IVF), intrauterine insemination (IUI), or intracytoplasmic sperm injection (ICSI) can assist conception.

- **Medications:** Fertility drugs to induce ovulation or regulate hormonal imbalances in conditions like PCOS.

- **Surgery:** Correcting anatomical issues, such as removing blockages or repairing reproductive organs, may improve fertility.

2. Lifestyle Modifications:

- **Healthy Diet and Exercise:** A balanced diet and regular exercise can improve overall health, which may positively impact fertility.

- **Weight Management:** Maintaining a healthy weight is crucial, as both underweight and overweight conditions can affect fertility.

- **Avoidance of Harmful Substances:** Limiting alcohol intake, avoiding smoking, and minimizing exposure to toxins can support fertility.

3. Alternative and Complementary Therapies:

- **Acupuncture:** Some studies suggest acupuncture may improve fertility outcomes by reducing stress and improving blood flow to reproductive organs.

- **Herbal Supplements:** Certain herbal supplements, like vitex or maca root, are believed to support hormonal balance and fertility, although evidence is limited.

4. **Assisted Reproduction Techniques:**

- **Egg or Sperm Donation:** In cases of severe infertility, using donor eggs or sperm can be an option.

- **Surrogacy:** In situations where carrying a pregnancy is not possible, surrogacy may be considered.

The Importance of Support and Patience:

Coping with fertility challenges requires patience,

resilience, and support. It's crucial to consult with healthcare professionals specializing in fertility, explore available options, and maintain open communication with partners.

Fertility challenges vary greatly among individuals, and what works for one person might not for another. A comprehensive approach, combining medical interventions, lifestyle adjustments, emotional support, and, if desired, alternative therapies, can help navigate and address fertility challenges while supporting overall well-being.

Exploring Infertility Causes

Infertility, defined as the inability to conceive after a year of regular, unprotected intercourse, can stem from various factors affecting both men and women. Understanding these causes is crucial in diagnosing and addressing fertility issues.

Female Factors:

1. **Ovulation Disorders:** Conditions like Polycystic Ovary Syndrome (PCOS), Primary Ovarian Insufficiency (POI), or hormonal imbalances can disrupt regular ovulation.

2. **Fallopian Tube Damage or Blockages:** Infections, endometriosis, or previous surgeries might affect the fallopian tubes, hindering the egg's journey to the uterus.

3. **Uterine Issues:** Structural abnormalities, fibroids, polyps, or scarring within the uterus can interfere with implantation.

4. **Age-related Decline in Egg Quality:** As women age, the quantity and quality of eggs decrease, impacting fertility.

Diagnostic Approaches:

1. **Medical History and Physical Exams:** Assessing medical history and conducting physical examinations to identify potential factors.

2. **Hormone Testing:** Assessing hormone levels to evaluate ovulation and reproductive health in both partners.

3. **Semen Analysis:** Evaluating sperm count, morphology, and motility in men.

4. **Imaging Tests:** Ultrasounds, hysterosalpingography, or laparoscopy to assess reproductive organs' structure and function.

5. **Genetic Testing:** Checking for genetic factors impacting fertility.

Treatment and Management:

The treatment of infertility depends on the identified cause. Options may include:

1. **Medications:** Hormonal therapies to regulate ovulation or improve sperm quality.

2. **Surgery:** Correcting structural issues in the reproductive system.

3. **Assisted Reproductive Technologies (ART):** Involving procedures like IVF, IUI, or ICSI.

4. **Lifestyle Changes:** Implementing healthy habits to improve fertility potential.

5. **Counseling and Support:** Emotional support and counseling can help cope with the challenges of infertility.

Exploring and understanding the causes of infertility is a critical step in developing tailored treatment plans to help couples achieve their goal of conceiving a child.

Holistic Remedies for Enhancing Fertility

Holistic approaches aim to address fertility by considering the interconnectedness of physical, emotional, and lifestyle factors. While they may not replace medical interventions, they can complement conventional treatments. Here are holistic remedies that might support fertility:

Diet and Nutrition:

1. **Balanced Diet:** Focus on whole, unprocessed foods rich in fruits, vegetables, lean proteins, healthy fats, and whole grains.

2. **Fertility-Boosting Foods:** Incorporate foods like leafy greens, berries, nuts, seeds, and oily fish that provide essential nutrients like antioxidants, omega-3 fatty acids, and vitamins important for fertility.

3. **Avoid Toxins:** Choose organic foods to minimize exposure to pesticides and hormones that might affect fertility.

Herbal Remedies:

1. **Chasteberry (Vitex):** Believed to help regulate hormones and promote ovulation.

2. **Maca Root:** Considered an adaptogen that might support hormone balance and fertility.

3. **Raspberry Leaf:** Known for its potential benefits for uterine health and fertility support.

Stress Management:

1. **Mindfulness and Relaxation:** Practices like yoga, meditation, or deep breathing exercises can reduce stress levels that might impact fertility.

2. **Acupuncture:** Some studies suggest that acupuncture may help manage stress and regulate reproductive hormones, potentially supporting fertility.

Lifestyle Adjustments:

1. **Maintain a Healthy Weight:** Both underweight and overweight conditions can impact fertility, so aim for a healthy BMI.

2. **Regular Exercise:** Engage in moderate physical activity, such as walking, swimming, or yoga, to support overall health and reduce stress.

3. **Adequate Sleep:** Prioritize quality sleep to support hormone regulation and overall well-being.

Environmental Considerations:

1. **Avoid Harmful Substances:** Limit exposure to environmental toxins, smoking, excessive alcohol, and caffeine, which might affect fertility.

2. **Reduce Chemical Exposure:** Use natural household and personal care products to minimize exposure to endocrine-disrupting chemicals.

Emotional Support and Relationships:

1. **Counseling and Support Groups:** Seek emotional support, whether through counseling or joining

support groups to navigate the emotional aspects of fertility struggles.

2. **Maintain Healthy Relationships:** Support from a partner or loved ones can positively impact emotional well-being during fertility challenges.

Holistic Approaches in Conjunction with Medical Care:

It's crucial to remember that while holistic remedies can complement conventional treatments, they should not replace medical advice or interventions. Consulting with healthcare professionals specializing in fertility can help develop a comprehensive plan that integrates holistic approaches with medical treatments to support fertility.

CHAPTER FOUR
Understanding Vaginitis

Vaginitis refers to inflammation of the vagina, often resulting from an imbalance or infection in the vaginal flora. It's a common condition that can cause discomfort and affect women of all ages. Understanding vaginitis involves recognizing its causes, symptoms, types, and available treatments.

Causes of Vaginitis:

1. **Bacterial Vaginosis (BV):** An imbalance in the normal bacteria of the vagina, characterized by an overgrowth of harmful bacteria.

2. **Yeast Infections:** Often caused by an overgrowth of the fungus Candida albicans, leading to symptoms like itching, burning, and abnormal discharge.

3. **Trichomoniasis:** A sexually transmitted infection (STI) caused by the parasite Trichomonas vaginalis, leading to vaginal irritation and discharge.

4. **Allergic Reactions:** Some women may experience vaginitis due to an allergic reaction to soaps, detergents, condoms, or other irritants.

5. **Hormonal Changes:** Changes in hormone levels, such as during pregnancy or menopause, can sometimes lead to vaginal irritation.

Symptoms of Vaginitis:

1. **Vaginal Discharge:** Changes in color, odor, or consistency of vaginal discharge.

2. **Itching or Irritation:** Vaginal itching or irritation, along with burning sensations during urination.

3. **Pain or Discomfort:** Painful intercourse or discomfort in the vaginal area.

4. **Redness or Swelling:** Swelling or redness in the vaginal area.

Types of Vaginitis:

1. **Bacterial Vaginosis (BV):** Characterized by a fishy-smelling discharge and often occurs due to an imbalance of bacteria.

2. **Yeast Infections:** Commonly identified by itching, burning, and a thick, white, cottage cheese-like discharge.

3. **Trichomoniasis:** Results in frothy, yellow-green vaginal discharge with a strong odor and vaginal irritation.

Diagnosis and Treatment:

1. **Medical Evaluation:** A healthcare provider may perform a pelvic exam and collect a vaginal sample for testing to diagnose the type of vaginitis.

2. **Medications:** Treatment varies depending on the cause and may include antibiotics, antifungal creams, or oral medications.

3. **Home Remedies:** For mild cases, over-the-counter antifungal or antibacterial creams may offer relief. Natural remedies like probiotics or herbal washes might also help.

4. **Avoiding Irritants:** Preventing further irritation by avoiding scented products, douches, or potential allergens.

5. **Partner Treatment:** For certain infections like trichomoniasis, partner treatment may be necessary to prevent reinfection.

Prevention:

1. **Good Hygiene:** Practice proper hygiene and avoid irritating products.

2. **Safe Sex:** Use condoms to reduce the risk of sexually transmitted infections.

3. **Avoiding Douching:** Douching can disrupt the natural balance of vaginal flora and increase the risk of vaginitis.

4. **Regular Check-ups:** Routine gynecological exams can help detect and address vaginitis early on.

Conclusion:

Understanding vaginitis involves recognizing its diverse

causes, symptoms, and available treatments. Seeking timely medical attention for proper diagnosis and treatment is crucial for effectively managing and alleviating discomfort associated with vaginitis.

Combatting Vaginitis Naturally

Combatting vaginitis, an inflammation of the vagina, naturally involves lifestyle changes and remedies that can help alleviate symptoms. However, it's essential to consult a healthcare provider to confirm the cause and ensure proper treatment. Natural approaches includes:

Maintaining Good Hygiene:

1. **Gentle Cleansing:** Use mild, unscented soaps or intimate washes to clean the vaginal area.

2. **Proper Hygiene Practices:** Wipe from front to back after using the bathroom to prevent the spread of bacteria from the anus to the vagina.

Probiotics:

1. **Yogurt:** Consuming yogurt containing live cultures with lactobacillus bacteria may help restore the natural balance of healthy bacteria in the vagina.

2. **Probiotic Supplements:** Consider probiotic supplements that specifically target vaginal health to promote a healthy vaginal microbiome.

Natural Remedies:

1. **Tea Tree Oil:** Diluted tea tree oil applied topically might have antimicrobial properties that could help with certain types of vaginitis. However, it's essential

to use it cautiously and dilute it properly to avoid irritation.

2. **Coconut Oil:** Applying coconut oil externally may help soothe irritation and provide some relief from discomfort.

Avoid Irritants:

1. **Avoid Harsh Products:** Steer clear of scented feminine hygiene products, harsh soaps, and perfumed or colored toilet paper that may cause irritation.

2. **Cotton Underwear:** Wear breathable, cotton underwear and avoid tight-fitting clothing to promote airflow and prevent moisture buildup.

Herbal Washes or Soaks:

1. **Herbal Soaks:** Taking a warm bath with soothing herbs like chamomile, calendula, or rosemary may help alleviate discomfort and inflammation.

2. **Herbal Washes:** Some people find relief by using herbal washes or rinses with ingredients like calendula or witch hazel.

Dietary Adjustments:

1. **Balanced Diet:** Eating a diet rich in fruits, vegetables, whole grains, and lean proteins can support overall health and immune function.

2. **Hydration:** Drink plenty of water to stay hydrated, which can help maintain vaginal moisture levels.

Prevention:

1. **Safe Sex Practices:** Using condoms can help prevent the spread of sexually transmitted infections (STIs) that can lead to vaginitis.

2. **Regular Check-ups:** Regular gynecological check-ups can help detect and address any issues early on.

Caution:

- Always consult a healthcare professional before using natural remedies, especially if you're unsure about their safety or if symptoms persist or worsen.

- Avoid self-diagnosis, especially with recurrent or persistent symptoms, as they could indicate an underlying condition requiring medical attention.

Natural remedies may provide relief for mild cases of vaginitis or as complementary support to conventional treatments. However, proper diagnosis and treatment guided by a healthcare provider remain essential for managing vaginitis effectively.

Natural Remedies and Self-Care Practices

Vaginitis, characterized by vaginal inflammation, discomfort, and abnormal discharge, can benefit from natural remedies and self-care practices that aim to alleviate symptoms and support vaginal health. Here are some holistic approaches:

Maintain Good Hygiene:

1. **Gentle Cleansing:** Use mild, unscented soaps or intimate washes to clean the vaginal area.

2. **Proper Hygiene:** Wipe from front to back after using the bathroom to prevent bacteria transfer from the anus to the vagina.

Probiotics:

1. **Probiotic-Rich Foods:** Incorporate yogurt with live cultures or kefir into your diet to support healthy vaginal flora.

2. **Probiotic Supplements:** Consider probiotic supplements specifically designed for vaginal health.

Herbal Remedies:

1. **Tea Tree Oil:** Diluted tea tree oil may have antimicrobial properties helpful for certain types of vaginitis. Use caution and dilute properly to avoid irritation.

2. **Coconut Oil:** Applying coconut oil externally may help soothe irritation and provide relief from discomfort.

Avoid Irritants:

1. **Scented Products:** Avoid scented feminine hygiene products, harsh soaps, and perfumed or colored toilet paper.

2. **Cotton Underwear:** Wear breathable, cotton underwear and avoid tight-fitting clothing to promote airflow and prevent moisture buildup.

Herbal Washes or Soaks:

1. **Herbal Baths:** Taking a warm bath with soothing herbs like chamomile, calendula, or rosemary may help alleviate discomfort and inflammation.

2. **Herbal Washes:** Some find relief using herbal washes or rinses with ingredients like calendula or witch hazel.

Dietary Adjustments:

1. **Balanced Diet:** Consume fruits, vegetables, whole grains, and lean proteins for overall health, which may indirectly support vaginal health.

2. **Hydration:** Stay well-hydrated to maintain vaginal moisture levels.

Avoiding Potential Triggers:

1. **Sexual Practices:** Be mindful of potential irritants during sexual activities, such as using condoms with non-irritating lubricants.

2. **Chemical Exposure:** Minimize exposure to harsh chemicals in personal care products that may irritate the vaginal area.

Caution and Consultation:

- Always consult a healthcare provider before using natural remedies, especially if you're uncertain about their safety or if symptoms persist or worsen.

- Avoid self-diagnosis, especially with recurrent or persistent symptoms, as they might indicate an underlying condition requiring medical attention.

Natural remedies and self-care practices can provide relief for mild cases of vaginitis or complement conventional treatments. However, proper diagnosis and treatment guided by a healthcare provider remain essential for managing vaginitis effectively.

CHAPTER FIVE
Understanding Fibroids

Fibroids, just like noncancerous growth is also known as "uterine leiomyomas", that grows in the uterus. They are quite common, with many women experiencing them at some point in their lives. Understanding fibroids involves recognizing their causes, symptoms, types, diagnosis, and available treatments.

Causes and Risk Factors:

1. **Hormonal Influence:** Estrogen and progesterone levels can promote the growth of fibroids.

2. **Genetic Predisposition:** Family history and genetic factors can contribute to their development.

3. **Hormonal Changes:** Pregnancy or perimenopause, when hormone levels fluctuate, can influence fibroid growth.

4. **Other Factors:** Obesity, early onset of menstruation, and vitamin D deficiency may also increase the risk.

Types of Fibroids:

1. **Intramural:** Located within the uterine wall, these are the most common type and may cause enlargement of the uterus.

2. **Submucosal:** Grow into the uterine cavity, potentially leading to heavy menstrual bleeding and fertility issues.

3. **Subserosa:** Develop on the outer uterine wall and might cause pressure on surrounding organs.

Symptoms:

1. **Menstrual Changes:** Heavy or prolonged menstrual bleeding, frequent periods, or spotting between periods.

2. **Pelvic Pain:** Discomfort or pain in the pelvis or lower back.

3. **Pressure or Enlargement:** Feeling of fullness or pressure in the pelvic area due to an enlarged uterus.

4. **Urinary or Bowel Issues:** Frequent urination or constipation due to fibroids pressing on adjacent organs.

5. **Fertility Issues:** Infertility or recurrent miscarriages in some cases.

Diagnosis:

1. **Physical Examination:** A pelvic exam to check for abnormalities or enlargement of the uterus.

2. **Imaging Tests:** Ultrasound, MRI, or other imaging techniques to visualize the size, number, and location of fibroids.

3. **Hysteroscopy or Biopsy:** Procedures to examine the uterine cavity or sample tissue for further evaluation in certain cases.

Treatment Options:

1. **Watchful Waiting:** Monitoring without treatment if fibroids are small, asymptomatic, or not affecting quality of life.

2. **Medications:** Hormonal birth control or other medications to regulate menstrual bleeding or reduce symptoms.

3. **Non-Invasive Procedures:** Options like uterine artery embolization or focused ultrasound surgery to shrink fibroids.

4. **Surgical Removal:** Myomectomy to remove fibroids while preserving the uterus or hysterectomy as a last

resort for severe cases or when fertility is not a concern.

Lifestyle and Self-Care:

1. **Healthy Diet:** Emphasize whole foods, fruits, vegetables, and lean proteins for overall health.

2. **Exercise:** Regular physical activity can help manage symptoms and promote well-being.

3. **Stress Management:** Techniques like meditation, yoga, or relaxation exercises to reduce stress.

Natural Approaches to Managing Fibroids

Natural approaches can complement traditional treatments in managing fibroids and alleviating symptoms. While they might not eliminate fibroids, they can help reduce symptoms and improve overall well-being. Here are some strategies:

Dietary Modifications:

1. **Anti-Inflammatory Diet:** Emphasize fruits, vegetables, whole grains, and healthy fats to reduce inflammation.

2. **Fiber-Rich Foods:** Increase intake of fiber to aid in estrogen metabolism and promote bowel regularity.

3. **Healthy Fats:** Include sources of omega-3 fatty acids like fish, flaxseeds, and walnuts to reduce inflammation.

Herbal Remedies:

1. **Chasteberry (Vitex):** Believed to help regulate hormone levels and reduce symptoms like heavy bleeding.

2. **Green Tea:** Contains antioxidants that might help reduce fibroid size and symptoms.

3. **Milk Thistle:** Some studies suggest it may help balance hormone levels.

Stress Management:

1. **Mindfulness and Relaxation Techniques:** Practices like yoga, meditation, or deep breathing exercises can help reduce stress.

2. **Adequate Sleep:** Prioritize good sleep to support hormonal balance and overall well-being.

Physical Activity:

1. **Regular Exercise:** Engage in moderate exercise, like walking or swimming, to help manage weight and reduce symptoms.

2. **Yoga or Pilates:** These practices can help relieve stress and improve flexibility.

Alternative Therapies:

1. **Acupuncture:** Some evidence suggests acupuncture might help manage pain and reduce fibroid size.

2. **Castor Oil Packs:** Applying warm castor oil packs to the abdomen may help reduce inflammation and improve circulation.

Supplements:

1. **Vitamin D:** Adequate levels of vitamin D might help regulate estrogen metabolism.

2. **Magnesium:** May help with muscle relaxation and alleviate cramping associated with fibroids.

Caution and Consultation:

- It's crucial to consult healthcare professionals before starting any new regimen or supplements, especially if you're considering herbal remedies or major dietary changes.

- Natural approaches can support symptom management but might not replace conventional medical treatments for fibroids.

Integrating these natural remedies and lifestyle changes into a comprehensive treatment plan, alongside medical interventions, when necessary, can potentially improve symptoms, reduce discomfort, and enhance overall quality of life for individuals with fibroids.

Tackling Fibroids Naturally

Tackling fibroids naturally involves adopting lifestyle changes and holistic approaches aimed at reducing symptoms, managing discomfort, and promoting overall well-being. While these methods may not eliminate fibroids entirely, they can help alleviate symptoms and support general health. Here are some natural strategies:

Diet and Nutrition:

1. **Anti-inflammatory Foods:** Emphasize a diet rich in fruits, vegetables, whole grains, and healthy fats to reduce inflammation associated with fibroids.

2. **Fiber-Rich Foods:** Opt for high-fiber foods like legumes, whole grains, and flaxseeds to support hormonal balance and bowel health.

3. **Lean Proteins:** Choose lean sources of protein like fish, chicken, and plant-based proteins to support overall health.

Herbal Remedies:

1. **Chasteberry (Vitex):** Believed to regulate hormone levels and potentially reduce symptoms like heavy bleeding and pain associated with fibroids.

2. **Turmeric:** Known for its anti-inflammatory properties, which might help manage inflammation related to fibroids.

3. **Ginger:** Can be used in teas or meals and may help alleviate pain and inflammation.

Stress Management:

1. **Mindfulness Practices:** Engage in relaxation techniques such as yoga, meditation, or deep breathing exercises to reduce stress levels.

2. **Adequate Sleep:** Prioritize quality sleep to support hormonal balance and overall well-being.

Exercise and Physical Activity:

1. **Regular Exercise:** Incorporate moderate exercise into your routine, such as walking, swimming, or cycling, to help manage weight and reduce symptoms.

2. **Yoga or Pilates:** These practices can aid in stress reduction and improve flexibility.

Heat Therapy:

1. **Warm Baths or Heating Pads:** Applying heat to the lower abdomen may help relieve discomfort and reduce muscle tension associated with fibroids.

Supplements:

1. **Vitamin D:** Adequate levels of vitamin D might aid in hormone regulation and overall health.

2. **Magnesium:** May help relax muscles and ease cramping associated with fibroids.

Regular Monitoring and Self-Care:

1. **Track Symptoms:** Keep a record of symptoms and their severity to monitor changes over time.

2. **Self-Care Practices:** Prioritize relaxation, engage in activities you enjoy, and maintain a positive mindset.

Consultation and Caution:

- Always consult healthcare professionals before starting any new supplements or making significant lifestyle changes, especially if you're considering herbal remedies.

- Natural approaches can complement conventional treatments but should not replace medical advice or prescribed treatments for fibroids.

By integrating these natural strategies into daily life, individuals with fibroids can potentially manage symptoms more effectively, improve overall health, and enhance their

quality of life.

CHAPTER SIX
Addressing Abnormal Uterine Bleeding

Abnormal Uterine Bleeding (AUB) can stem from various factors, including hormonal imbalances, uterine fibroids, polyps, endometriosis, pelvic inflammatory disease (PID), thyroid disorders, or certain medications.

Symptoms: Irregular menstrual cycles, heavy or prolonged bleeding, bleeding between periods, or bleeding after menopause are common indicators of AUB.

Diagnosis and Evaluation:

1. **Medical History and Physical Exam:** Assessing medical history, including menstrual patterns, and performing a pelvic exam to identify potential causes.

2. **Blood Tests:** Assessing hormone levels, thyroid function, and blood clotting factors to determine underlying issues.

3. **Ultrasound or Imaging:** Visualizing the uterus and ovaries through imaging tests to detect abnormalities such as fibroids, polyps, or structural issues.

4. **Biopsy or Hysteroscopy:** Sampling uterine tissue or using a small camera to examine the uterus and detect any abnormalities.

Treatment Approaches:

1. **Hormonal Therapy:** Birth control pills, hormonal IUDs, or hormone therapies to regulate menstrual cycles and reduce bleeding.

2. **Non-Hormonal Medications:** Tranexamic acid or NSAIDs (Nonsteroidal Anti-Inflammatory Drugs) to reduce heavy bleeding.

3. **Intrauterine Procedures:** Endometrial ablation or a hysterectomy for severe cases or when other treatments fail.

4. **Fertility Treatments:** Addressing underlying issues affecting fertility in cases were abnormal bleeding impacts conception.

Lifestyle Adjustments:

1. **Healthy Diet:** Incorporating nutrient-rich foods to support overall health and hormone balance.

2. **Regular Exercise:** Engaging in regular physical activity to maintain a healthy weight and improve overall well-being.

3. **Stress Management:** Practicing relaxation techniques like yoga, meditation, or deep breathing to reduce stress levels.

Caution and Consultation:

- It's crucial to consult with healthcare professionals to determine the cause of abnormal bleeding and appropriate treatment options.

- Addressing abnormal uterine bleeding requires proper diagnosis and personalized treatment plans tailored to individual needs.

- Lifestyle changes and natural remedies can complement medical treatments but should not replace professional medical advice or prescribed treatments for abnormal uterine bleeding.

By understanding the potential causes, seeking timely

medical evaluation, and exploring appropriate treatments, individuals experiencing abnormal uterine bleeding can manage their symptoms effectively and improve their quality of life.

Understanding Causes of Uterine Bleeding

Understanding the causes of uterine bleeding is a crucial step towards empowering women with knowledge about their health. Uterine bleeding, often irregular or abnormal, can be a perplexing occurrence, eliciting concern and uncertainty. Delving into its multifaceted causes unravels a spectrum of factors contributing to this phenomenon:

Hormonal Imbalances:

1. **Menstrual Cycle Disruptions:** Fluctuations in estrogen and progesterone levels can result in irregular bleeding patterns.

2. **Perimenopause and Menopause:** Hormonal shifts during these life phases can lead to unpredictable bleeding.

Structural Issues:

1. **Uterine Fibroids:** Non-cancerous growths in the uterine wall can cause heavy, prolonged bleeding or spotting.

2. **Polyps:** Overgrowths of tissue in the uterus can trigger irregular bleeding.

3. **Adenomyosis:** When the uterine lining grows into the muscle wall, it can cause heavy or prolonged bleeding.

Medical Conditions:

1. **Endometriosis:** The presence of endometrial tissue outside the uterus can result in abnormal bleeding.

2. **Pelvic Inflammatory Disease (PID):** Infections in the reproductive organs may cause irregular bleeding.

3. **Thyroid Disorders:** Imbalances in thyroid hormones can impact menstrual cycles and lead to abnormal bleeding.

Medications and Health Factors:

1. **Blood Thinners:** Certain medications affect blood clotting and may cause increased bleeding.

2. **Stress and Lifestyle Factors:** High stress levels or drastic changes in weight or exercise routines might disrupt menstrual cycles.

Pregnancy-Related Causes:

1. **Ectopic Pregnancy:** A pregnancy outside the uterus can cause vaginal bleeding and severe abdominal pain.

2. **Miscarriage or Pregnancy Complications:** Bleeding during pregnancy might indicate complications needing immediate medical attention.

Cancerous Conditions:

1. **Endometrial Cancer:** Irregular bleeding, especially after menopause, could be a symptom.

2. **Cervical or Uterine Cancer:** Unusual bleeding, pain, or discomfort might signal a serious issue.

Diagnosis and Management:

Understanding the cause of uterine bleeding often involves a comprehensive evaluation, including medical history, physical exams, blood tests, imaging studies like ultrasounds, and sometimes biopsies. Management varies based on the underlying cause, ranging from hormonal therapies to surgeries or lifestyle adjustments.

Seeking Medical Guidance:

It's crucial to consult healthcare professionals when experiencing abnormal uterine bleeding. Open communication, timely evaluations, and appropriate treatments not only address the immediate concerns but also promote overall health and well-being.

Understanding the intricate web of factors contributing to uterine bleeding empowers women to advocate for their health, seek appropriate care, and embark on a journey towards informed decisions and better reproductive health outcomes.

Natural Remedies and Lifestyle Changes

Addressing uterine bleeding through natural remedies and lifestyle changes involves holistic approaches aimed at alleviating symptoms and promoting overall health. Here's an exploration of these methods:

Herbal Remedies:

1. **Chasteberry (Vitex):** Known for hormonal balance, potentially regulating menstrual cycles and reducing heavy bleeding.

2. **Raspberry Leaf:** May tone the uterus and reduce heavy bleeding.

Dietary Adjustments:

1. **Iron-Rich Foods:** Incorporate spinach, lentils, and fortified cereals to combat iron loss due to heavy bleeding.

2. **Omega-3 Fatty Acids:** Found in fatty fish, flaxseeds, and walnuts, they may reduce inflammation and menstrual discomfort.

Herbs and Supplements:

1. **Evening Primrose Oil:** Contains omega-6 fatty acids, potentially reducing menstrual cramps and heavy bleeding.

2. **Dong Quai:** Often used in traditional Chinese medicine to regulate menstrual cycles and reduce bleeding.

Lifestyle Changes:

1. **Regular Exercise:** Engage in moderate exercise like walking or yoga to improve circulation and manage stress, potentially aiding in menstrual regulation.

2. **Stress Management:** Practices like meditation, deep breathing, or yoga can help reduce stress, which might impact menstrual irregularities.

Hydration and Sleep:

1. **Adequate Hydration:** Ensure sufficient water intake to maintain overall health and aid in bodily functions.

2. **Quality Sleep:** Aim for a consistent sleep schedule and create a relaxing bedtime routine to support hormonal balance.

Healthy Practices:

1. **Limit Caffeine and Alcohol:** Both can exacerbate hormonal imbalances and contribute to irregular bleeding.

2. **Quit Smoking:** Smoking can impact hormonal levels and worsen menstrual irregularities.

Caution and Consultation:

- Natural remedies should be used cautiously and under the guidance of healthcare professionals, especially if other medical conditions or medications are involved.

- Lifestyle changes, while beneficial, should complement professional medical advice and treatments, not replace them.

Integrating these natural remedies and lifestyle changes can contribute to managing uterine bleeding and improving overall well-being. However, individual responses vary, and seeking guidance from healthcare providers ensures personalized and comprehensive care.

CHAPTER SEVEN
Understanding Endometriosis

Understanding endometriosis involves grasping a complex condition that affects individuals with a uterus. Endometriosis occurs when tissue similar to the lining of the uterus grows outside the uterus, causing pain, inflammation, and potential fertility issues.

Firstly, comprehending the symptoms is crucial. Women with endometriosis often experience pelvic pain, painful periods, heavy bleeding, pain during intercourse, and sometimes, difficulty conceiving. However, symptoms can vary widely among individuals, making diagnosis challenging.

The diagnostic process typically involves a combination of medical history evaluation, pelvic exams, imaging tests like ultrasounds, and sometimes laparoscopic surgery for a definitive diagnosis. Early detection is key, but unfortunately, it often takes years for individuals to receive an accurate diagnosis due to the similarity of symptoms to other conditions and the lack of awareness.

Understanding the impact of endometriosis on one's life is vital. The chronic pain and associated symptoms can significantly affect mental health, relationships, work, and daily activities. Managing these effects often requires a multidisciplinary approach involving gynecologists, pain specialists, mental health professionals, and sometimes, fertility experts.

Treatment options vary based on the severity of symptoms and the individual's goals. They may include pain management through medications, hormonal therapies, lifestyle changes, or surgery to remove the endometrial tissue. While there's no cure, proper management can significantly improve quality of life.

Raising awareness about endometriosis is essential. Education about the condition can lead to earlier diagnosis, improved support for affected individuals, and better understanding among the general population. Advocacy efforts push for increased research funding, improved healthcare access, and better treatment options for those impacted by this condition.

Empathy and support play crucial roles in helping individuals with endometriosis navigate their journey. Understanding their experiences, offering support, and advocating for better healthcare resources can make a significant difference in their lives.

Managing Endometriosis Holistically

Managing endometriosis holistically involves a

comprehensive approach that addresses not only the physical symptoms but also the mental, emotional, and lifestyle aspects of the condition. Here are some holistic strategies that individuals with endometriosis often find beneficial:

1. **Nutrition:** Adopting an anti-inflammatory diet can help reduce inflammation associated with endometriosis. This includes incorporating whole foods, fruits, vegetables, omega-3 fatty acids (found in fish, flaxseeds, and walnuts), and minimizing processed foods, caffeine, and alcohol.

2. **Exercise and Movement:** Regular physical activity can help alleviate pain and improve overall well-being. Low-impact exercises like swimming, yoga, or walking is very essential to the general wellbeing.

3. **Stress Management:** Stress can exacerbate symptoms. Techniques like mindfulness meditation, deep breathing exercises, or engaging in hobbies and activities that promote relaxation can help manage stress levels.

4. **Alternative Therapies:** Some individuals find relief through acupuncture, chiropractic care, or herbal supplements. However, it's crucial to consult with healthcare providers before trying any alternative therapies to ensure they complement the treatment plan.

5. **Pain Management Techniques:** Heat therapy (using heating pads or warm baths) and transcutaneous electrical nerve stimulation (TENS) units can help manage pain without relying solely on medication.

6. **Hormonal Balance:** Hormonal treatments such as birth control pills or other hormone therapies can help regulate menstrual cycles and reduce pain. However, these should be discussed with healthcare providers to understand their potential benefits and risks.

7. **Support Networks:** Joining support groups or seeking counseling can provide emotional support and practical advice from others who understand the challenges of living with endometriosis.

8. **Regular Monitoring and Communication:** It's essential to have regular check-ups with healthcare providers and maintain open communication about the effectiveness of treatment strategies.

9. **Lifestyle Adjustments:** Understanding personal triggers that exacerbate symptoms, such as certain

foods or environmental factors, and making lifestyle adjustments accordingly can significantly impact symptom management.

10. **Holistic Healthcare Team:** Building a team of healthcare professionals—including gynecologists, nutritionists, physical therapists, mental health specialists, and alternative medicine practitioners—can provide a comprehensive approach to managing endometriosis.

Holistic management focuses on addressing the individual's overall well-being, acknowledging that the impact of endometriosis goes beyond physical symptoms. It's crucial for individuals to work closely with their healthcare team to develop a personalized holistic plan that suits their specific needs and preferences.

Natural Strategies For Alleviating Symptoms

Managing endometriosis symptoms naturally involves various approaches that aim to reduce pain, inflammation, and overall discomfort associated with the condition. While these methods may not cure endometriosis, they can help alleviate symptoms and improve quality of life for some individuals. Here's a comprehensive overview:

1. **Dietary Modifications:**

   - **Anti-Inflammatory Diet:** Emphasize whole, nutrient-dense foods like fruits, vegetables, whole grains, and lean proteins. Omega-3 fatty acids found in fish, flaxseeds, and walnuts have anti-inflammatory properties and may help reduce pain.

   - **Avoid Trigger Foods:** Limiting or avoiding inflammatory foods such as processed foods, red meat, dairy, caffeine, and alcohol might help reduce inflammation and alleviate symptoms.

2. **Herbal Supplements:**

- **Turmeric and Ginger:** These herbs possess anti-inflammatory properties that may help reduce pain and inflammation. Chamomile tea might also provide soothing effects.

- **Consultation is Key:** It's crucial to consult with healthcare professionals before incorporating herbal supplements to ensure they're safe and won't interfere with prescribed medications.

3. **Heat Therapy:**

- Applying heat to the lower abdomen using heating pads or warm baths can help relax pelvic muscles, alleviate cramping, and reduce pain associated with endometriosis.

4. Acupuncture:

- This traditional Chinese practice involves inserting thin needles into specific points in the body to alleviate pain and promote overall well-being. Some individuals find relief from endometriosis symptoms through acupuncture.

5. Exercise and Movement:

- Regular physical activity, such as yoga, Pilates, stretching, or low-impact exercises, can improve circulation, reduce stress, and potentially alleviate pain associated with endometriosis.

6. Mindfulness and Stress Reduction:

- Mindfulness meditation, deep breathing exercises, tai chi, and yoga can help manage stress levels. Stress reduction techniques may help alleviate symptoms aggravated by stress.

7. Aromatherapy:

- Essential oils like lavender, peppermint, or clary sage might offer relaxation and pain relief when used through aromatherapy or diluted application. However, individual responses may vary.

8. Chiropractic Care:

- Spinal adjustments or chiropractic treatments might help alleviate pelvic pain by addressing misalignments and reducing tension in the pelvic region.

9. Pelvic Floor Physical Therapy:

- Working with a pelvic floor physical therapist can help address muscle tension and dysfunction in the pelvic area, potentially reducing pain and discomfort.

10. Support and Education:

- Joining support groups, seeking guidance from healthcare professionals, and educating oneself about the condition can empower individuals to better manage their symptoms and advocate for their healthcare needs.

CHAPTER EIGHT
Understanding Cervical Cancer

Cervical cancer is a significant health concern worldwide, impacting millions of lives each year. Understanding its causes, risk factors, detection, and prevention is crucial in combatting this disease.

At its core, cervical cancer develops in the cervix, the lower part of the uterus that connects to the vagina. The primary cause is the human papillomavirus (HPV), a common sexually transmitted infection. Certain strains of the virus, especially HPV 16 and 18, pose a higher risk.

Risk factors for cervical cancer include early sexual activity, multiple sexual partners, a weakened immune system, smoking, long-term use of oral contraceptives, and a family history of the disease. However, it's important to note that anyone with a cervix can develop cervical cancer, regardless of their risk factors.

Regular screenings, particularly Pap tests and HPV tests, are vital for early detection. Pap tests involve collecting cells from the cervix to identify any abnormal changes. HPV tests specifically look for the presence of the virus. Early detection significantly improves treatment outcomes, as cervical cancer is highly treatable in its early stages.

The choice of treatment is personalized and considers factors like the stage of cancer, overall health, and patient preferences.

Prevention plays a pivotal role in reducing the incidence of cervical cancer. Vaccination against HPV significantly lowers the risk of infection with high-risk strains. The HPV vaccine is recommended for both girls and boys before they become sexually active, typically around ages 11-12. However, it can still be effective when administered later.

Regular screenings, practicing safe sex, limiting sexual partners, quitting smoking, and maintaining a healthy lifestyle to boost the immune system all contribute to reducing the risk of cervical cancer.

Education and awareness are essential in the fight against cervical cancer. Promoting access to healthcare, especially in underserved communities, and providing accurate information about prevention and early detection are critical steps in reducing the burden of this disease.

Understanding cervical cancer involves knowing its causes, risk factors, detection methods, treatment options, and prevention strategies. With a comprehensive approach that encompasses education, vaccination, screenings, and healthcare accessibility, we can make significant strides in reducing the prevalence and impact of cervical cancer globally.

Awareness And Prevention Of Cervical Cancer

Raising awareness and emphasizing prevention strategies are pivotal in the fight against cervical cancer. Below are precise exploration of these aspects:

Awareness Campaigns:

1. **Education Initiatives:** Comprehensive campaigns should educate individuals about cervical cancer, its risk factors, and the importance of regular screenings.

2. **Targeted Outreach:** Tailored efforts should reach communities with limited access to healthcare or knowledge about cervical cancer.

3. **Media and Publicity:** Utilizing various media platforms to disseminate accurate information, debunk myths, and encourage preventive actions can significantly impact public awareness.

Prevention Strategies:

1. **HPV Vaccination:** Encouraging vaccination against HPV for both genders before exposure to the virus is crucial. Increasing accessibility and affordability of vaccines is vital.

2. **Regular Screenings:** Promoting routine Pap tests and HPV tests for early detection among women aged 21-65 can significantly reduce the incidence of advanced-stage cervical cancer.

3. **Safe Sexual Practices:** Advocating for safe sex practices, including condom use, limiting sexual partners, and discussing sexual health openly, helps prevent HPV transmission.

4. **Smoking Cessation Programs:** Highlighting the link between smoking and cervical cancer and

providing support for quitting smoking can lower risk factors.

Accessible Healthcare:

1. **Healthcare Equity:** Ensuring access to affordable healthcare services, especially in underserved communities, is crucial for early detection and treatment.

2. **Screening Programs:** Establishing and promoting government-sponsored or community-based screening programs can reach a larger population.

3. **Support and Counseling:** Providing psychological support and counseling for individuals diagnosed with HPV or cervical cancer is essential for their well-being and adherence to treatment.

Community Engagement:

1. **Support Groups:** Creating support networks and groups for cervical cancer survivors and patients fosters emotional support and shared experiences.

2. **Cultural Sensitivity:** Tailoring awareness programs to address cultural beliefs and practices regarding health and reproductive issues is crucial for community acceptance and participation.

3. **Peer Education:** Engaging peer educators or community health workers to disseminate information within their communities can enhance understanding and trust.

Continued Research:

1. **Innovative Approaches:** Investing in research for better diagnostic tools, treatment methods, and

understanding the HPV virus can improve prevention and treatment outcomes.

2. **Global Collaboration:** International partnerships can facilitate sharing knowledge, resources, and best practices, benefiting populations globally.

By combining comprehensive awareness campaigns, effective prevention strategies, accessible healthcare, community engagement, and continued research efforts, we can significantly reduce the incidence of cervical cancer and save lives worldwide.

Natural Supportive Measures And Prevention

Natural supportive measures and preventive strategies play a significant role in reducing the risk of cervical cancer. While these methods are not standalone treatments, they can complement conventional medical approaches. Here's an exploration of these supportive measures:

Dietary Changes:

1. **Antioxidant-Rich Foods:** Consuming a diet abundant in fruits and vegetables, particularly those rich in antioxidants like beta-carotene, vitamin C, and vitamin E, may help combat cellular damage caused by free radicals.

2. **Cruciferous Vegetables:** Incorporating broccoli, cauliflower, kale, and Brussels sprouts, known for their sulfur-containing compounds, can potentially assist in detoxification processes and lower cancer risk.

3. **Healthy Fats:** Including sources of omega-3 fatty acids like flaxseeds, chia seeds, and fatty fish may

have anti-inflammatory properties, supporting overall health.

Herbal Supplements:

1. **Green Tea Extract:** Studies suggest that compounds in green tea, such as catechins, possess anti-cancer properties and may contribute to reducing the risk of cervical cancer.

2. **Turmeric/Curcumin:** Curcumin, the active ingredient in turmeric, has shown anti-inflammatory and anti-cancer effects in various studies and may aid in preventing cancer development.

3. **Astragalus Root:** Known for its immune-boosting properties, astragalus may support the immune system in fighting infections, potentially reducing HPV persistence.

Lifestyle Modifications:

1. **Regular Exercise:** Engaging in regular physical activity not only supports overall health but also contributes to a stronger immune system and reduced inflammation, potentially lowering cancer risk.

2. **Stress Reduction Techniques:** Chronic stress can weaken the immune system. Practices like meditation, yoga, or mindfulness may aid in stress reduction and support overall well-being.

3. **Adequate Sleep:** Prioritizing good sleep hygiene is essential, as quality sleep supports immune function and overall health.

Natural Hygiene Practices:

1. **Maintaining Vaginal Health:** Practices like using gentle, unscented soaps, avoiding douching, and

wearing breathable underwear can help maintain a healthy vaginal environment.

2. **Regular Hydration:** Staying well-hydrated supports overall health and aids in maintaining optimal bodily functions, including immune response.

Regular Screening and Monitoring:

Natural measures should complement, not replace, regular screenings and medical consultations. Despite incorporating natural supportive measures, routine screenings for cervical cancer and HPV testing remain crucial for early detection and timely intervention. In conclusion, it is essential to consult healthcare professionals before starting any new supplements or making significant lifestyle changes, especially if diagnosed with HPV or cervical abnormalities. Natural supportive measures are not a substitute for medical treatment and should be used in conjunction with professional medical advice and treatments.

By incorporating these natural supportive measures alongside conventional preventive strategies, individuals can potentially reduce their risk of cervical cancer and promote overall health and well-being.

CHAPTER NINE
Understanding Interstitial Cystitis

Interstitial Cystitis (IC), also known as painful bladder syndrome, is a chronic condition affecting the bladder. It's characterized by discomfort, pressure, or pain in the bladder and pelvic region. Understanding this condition involves delving into its symptoms, potential causes, diagnosis, and management strategies.

Symptoms:

1. **Pelvic Pain:** Persistent discomfort or pain in the pelvic region, often worsening as the bladder fills.

2. **Urinary Urgency and Frequency:** Frequent, urgent needs to urinate, even when the bladder contains minimal urine.

3. **Pain during Intercourse:** Some individuals may experience pain or discomfort during sexual intercourse.

4. **Nocturia:** Waking up multiple times during the night to urinate.

5. **Symptoms Variability:** Symptoms may vary over time, with periods of remission and flare-ups.

Potential Causes:

The exact cause of IC remains unclear, but several factors may contribute:

- **Bladder Lining Defects:** Damage to the bladder lining, allowing irritating substances in urine to penetrate deeper layers.

- **Immune System Abnormalities:** An autoimmune response targeting the bladder.

- **Neurological Factors:** Issues with nerve signaling leading to increased sensation of pain.

- **Pelvic Floor Dysfunction:** Problems with the muscles and tissues surrounding the bladder.

Diagnosis:

Diagnosing IC involves ruling out other conditions with similar symptoms:

- **Medical History and Physical Examination:** Detailed discussions about symptoms and a physical examination.

- **Urinalysis and Culture:** To rule out urinary tract infections (UTIs) or other urinary disorders.

- **Cystoscopy:** A procedure to examine the bladder using a thin tube with a camera (cystoscope).

- **Biopsy:** In some cases, a biopsy of the bladder lining may be performed.

Management and Treatment:

1. **Lifestyle Changes:** Avoiding bladder irritants like caffeine, acidic foods, alcohol, and artificial sweeteners. Keeping up with a healthy diet lifestyle managing your stress level can help in relieving these symptoms.

2. **Medications:** Prescription medications such as oral medications to reduce bladder inflammation or bladder installations (medications directly introduced into the bladder).

3. **Physical Therapy:** Pelvic floor exercises or physical therapy to relax and strengthen pelvic floor muscles.

4. **Nerve Stimulation:** Techniques like sacral neuromodulation may help modulate nerve activity.

5. **Bladder Distention:** In some cases, stretching the bladder during cystoscopy may provide temporary relief.

Living with IC can be challenging. Support groups, counseling, or therapy may aid in coping with the emotional and psychological impact of the condition. Managing stress and finding ways to relax can also improve symptoms.

Conclusion:

Understanding interstitial cystitis involves recognizing its chronic nature and the impact it has on individuals' daily lives. While there's no definitive cure, a multidisciplinary approach focusing on symptom management, lifestyle adjustments, and personalized treatments can significantly improve the quality of life for those affected by this condition.

Coping With Interstitial Cystitis

Coping with Interstitial Cystitis (IC) can be challenging due to its chronic and often unpredictable nature. Here's a guide on managing and coping with IC:

Education and Understanding:

1. **Learn About IC:** Educating yourself about the condition helps you understand its symptoms, triggers, and available treatments.

2. **Consult Healthcare Professionals:** Regular communication with healthcare providers ensures access to the latest information and personalized treatment options.

Lifestyle Adjustments:

1. **Dietary Modifications:** Identify and avoid foods or drinks that trigger symptoms. Common triggers

include caffeine, alcohol, acidic foods, and artificial sweeteners.

2. **Hydration:** Maintain adequate hydration without overloading the bladder.

3. **Bladder Health:** Practice good bladder habits, such as urinating when needed and avoiding holding urine for too long.

Stress Management:

1. **Stress Reduction Techniques:** Explore stress-relief methods like meditation, deep breathing exercises, yoga, or mindfulness to manage stress, which can exacerbate IC symptoms.

2. **Relaxation Techniques:** Engage in activities that promote relaxation, such as reading, listening to music, taking warm baths, or hobbies that bring joy.

Pain Management:

1. **Heat Therapy:** Applying heat to the pelvic area or taking warm baths can alleviate discomfort.

2. **Prescribed Medications:** Discuss with healthcare providers about medications to manage pain or reduce bladder inflammation.

3. **Physical Therapy:** Pelvic floor physical therapy may assist in relieving pelvic pain or discomfort.

Support Networks:

1. **Join Support Groups:** Connecting with others who have IC provides emotional support, shared experiences, and practical advice.

2. **Therapy or Counseling:** Seek professional help to navigate the emotional impact of living with a chronic condition and learn coping strategies.

Self-Care and Mindfulness:

1. **Prioritize Self-Care:** Maintain a healthy lifestyle, including adequate sleep, regular exercise, and a balanced diet to support overall well-being.

2. **Mindfulness Practices:** Practice self-compassion and mindfulness to accept and manage the challenges that come with IC.

Communication:

1. **Open Communication:** Communicate openly with family, friends, and employers about your condition and needs.

2. **Work Accommodations:** Discuss workplace accommodations with employers if needed, such as flexible schedules or ergonomic adjustments.

Patience and Positivity:

1. **Be Patient:** Managing IC is a journey that may require time and adjustments. Celebrate small victories along the way.

2. **Stay Positive:** Focus on activities and aspects of life that bring joy and fulfillment.

Conclusion:

Coping with Interstitial Cystitis involves a multifaceted approach that combines education, lifestyle adjustments, stress management, seeking support, and practicing self-care. While there's no one-size-fits-all solution, a personalized and holistic approach can significantly improve the quality of life for individuals living with IC.

Natural Approaches For Relief

Natural approaches for relieving Interstitial Cystitis (IC) symptoms often complement medical treatments. These methods aim to alleviate discomfort and manage symptoms through natural means:

Dietary Modifications:

1. **Bladder-Friendly Diet:** Identify and eliminate potential trigger foods like caffeine, spicy foods, acidic fruits, alcohol, and artificial sweeteners.

2. **Hydration:** Drink water regularly to maintain hydration without overloading the bladder. Limiting intake of bladder irritants like carbonated drinks can also help.

Supplements and Herbs:

1. **Quercetin:** This antioxidant may have anti-inflammatory properties, potentially aiding in reducing bladder inflammation.

2. **Marshmallow Root:** Known for its soothing properties, it might provide relief by coating and protecting the bladder lining.

3. **Aloe Vera:** Some individuals find relief from aloe vera juice, believed to have anti-inflammatory effects.

Bladder Support:

1. **Heat Therapy:** Applying a heating pad or warm compress to the pelvic area may ease discomfort and relax pelvic muscles.

2. **Herbal Teas:** Chamomile or peppermint teas are often considered soothing and might provide mild relief.

Stress Management:

1. **Mindfulness and Relaxation Techniques:** Practices like deep breathing exercises, meditation, yoga, or tai chi can help manage stress, which often exacerbates IC symptoms.

2. **Biofeedback:** Learning techniques to control body responses to stress might assist in managing pelvic floor muscle tension.

Physical Therapy:

1. **Pelvic Floor Exercises:** Working with a physical therapist to strengthen and relax pelvic floor muscles may alleviate symptoms.

2. **Bladder Retraining:** Techniques to control and manage urination frequency can be taught by specialized therapists.

Alternative Therapies:

1. **Acupuncture:** Some individuals report relief from IC symptoms through acupuncture, believed to restore balance and relieve pain.

2. **Essential Oils:** Certain oils like lavender or chamomile, when diluted and used in baths or for massage, might provide relaxation and alleviate discomfort.

Probiotics:

1. **Lactobacillus:** Some research suggests that certain probiotics might aid in restoring healthy bacteria in the gut and urinary tract, potentially reducing inflammation.

Lifestyle Adjustments:

1. **Avoiding Irritants:** Use unscented, gentle hygiene products, and avoid tight-fitting clothing that may irritate the pelvic area.

2. **Bladder Emptying Techniques:** Ensure complete emptying of the bladder when urinating, leaning forward or using relaxation techniques may help.

Caution and Consultation:

- Always consult healthcare professionals before starting any new supplements, herbs, or alternative therapies, especially if on medications or diagnosed with IC.

- Natural approaches should complement, not replace, medical treatments. It's crucial to work with healthcare providers to devise a holistic approach to manage IC symptoms effectively.

Natural approaches for IC management vary from person to person, so it's essential to explore and discover what works best for individual needs. Integrating these natural methods into a comprehensive treatment plan may offer relief and improve overall quality of life for those living with IC.

Embracing Natural Healing For Female Reproductive Health

Embracing natural healing for female reproductive health involves holistic approaches that support and nurture the body's natural functions. Here's an exploration of practices and methods:

Nutrition and Diet:

1. **Balanced Diet:** Emphasize whole foods, fruits, vegetables, lean proteins, and healthy fats to support overall health.

2. **Specific Nutrients:** Incorporate foods rich in iron, calcium, omega-3 fatty acids, and antioxidants to support reproductive health.

Herbal Remedies:

1. **Chasteberry:** Known for hormonal balance support, potentially aiding menstrual irregularities and premenstrual symptoms.

2. **Red Raspberry Leaf:** Often used to tone the uterus and support menstrual health.

3. **Nettle Leaf:** Contains nutrients beneficial for hormonal balance and may alleviate menstrual cramps.

Stress Management:

1. **Mindfulness Practices:** Meditation, yoga, deep breathing exercises, or tai chi can help manage stress, supporting hormone balance.

2. **Therapeutic Activities:** Engage in hobbies, creative pursuits, or activities that promote relaxation and reduce stress.

Hormonal Balance:

1. **Seed Cycling:** Consuming specific seeds (flaxseeds, pumpkin seeds, sunflower seeds, and sesame seeds) during different phases of the menstrual cycle to support hormonal balance.

2. **Balanced Exercise:** Regular, moderate exercise can aid in hormone regulation and overall well-being.

Menstrual Health:

1. **Menstrual Hygiene Products:** Consider natural or organic alternatives like menstrual cups or cloth pads to reduce exposure to chemicals.

2. **Healthy Practices:** Adequate rest, hydration, and heat therapy (using heating pads) can help manage menstrual discomfort.

Fertility Support:

1. **Fertility Awareness Methods:** Tracking basal body temperature, cervical mucus, and menstrual cycles to aid in understanding ovulation patterns.

2. **Nutritional Support:** Ensuring adequate intake of fertility-supporting nutrients like folic acid, zinc, and vitamin D.

Holistic Practices:

1. **Acupuncture:** Some women find acupuncture helpful for regulating menstrual cycles and reducing stress, supporting reproductive health.

2. **Aromatherapy:** Using essential oils like clary sage or lavender in diluted forms for relaxation and hormone balance.

Communication and Regular Check-Ups:

1. **Open Dialogue:** Discuss concerns or changes in menstrual cycles, reproductive health, or fertility with healthcare providers.

2. **Regular Screenings:** Schedule routine gynecological exams and screenings to monitor reproductive health.

Caution and Consultation:

- Prioritize safety and consult healthcare providers before incorporating new herbs, supplements, or alternative therapies, especially if pregnant, breastfeeding, or dealing with specific health conditions.

- Natural approaches should complement, not replace, medical advice or treatments for reproductive health issues.

By embracing natural healing methods alongside traditional medical care, women can support their reproductive health holistically. Personalized approaches catered to individual needs and in conjunction with professional guidance can enhance overall well-being and empower women to take charge of their reproductive health.

About The Book

This book titled, "Natural Remedy 4 Female Reproductive System Disorders" was written by Mrs. Vera Jacob who is a naturalist, herbalist, and an astute student of the late Dr. Sebi. In this guide, Mrs. Jacob will walk you through a step-by-step process on how to prevent, manage, and treat all forms of female reproductive system disorders such as; Infertility, PCOS, POI, Endometriosis, Abnormal Uterine Bleeding, Interstitial Cystitis (IC), Vaginitis, Fibroids, Cervical Cancer, menstrual irregularities, hormonal imbalances, menopause, etc., naturally without the fear of any possible side effect.

The book aims to empower women by providing accessible and natural methods to prevent, manage, and treat all types of female reproductive system disorders, balancing physical, emotional, and mental well-being and a lot more.